# Chair Yoga

## Easy, Healing Moves You Can Do with a Chair

## Blythe Ayne, PhD

# *Chair Yoga –*
## *Easy, Healing Moves You Can Do With a Chair*
### *Blythe Ayne, Ph.D.*

### *Emerson & Tilman, Publishers*
129 Pendleton Way #55
Washougal, WA 98671

Book, drawings, & cover design by Blythe Ayne
Text & Drawings © Blythe Ayne
*Thank you C. Greear for your stellar editing*

Other books in the *Absolute Beginner* series:
*Bed Yoga – Easy, Healing, Yoga Moves You Can Do in Bed*
*Bed Yoga for Couples—Easy, Healing, Yoga Moves You Can Do in Bed*
*Write Your Book! Publish Your Book! Market Your Book!*

*www.BlytheAyne.com*

ebook ISBN: 978-1-957272–57-3
Paperback ISBN: 978-1-957272-56-6
Hardbound ISBN: 978-1-957272-58-0
Large Print ISBN: 978-1-957272-59-7

[1. HEALTH & FITNESS/Diet & Nutrition/Yoga
2. HEALTH & FITNESS/Healing
3. BODY, MIND & SPIRIT/Healing/Energy]
BIC: FM
First Edition

# Chair Yoga

## Easy, Healing Moves You Can Do with a Chair

## Blythe Ayne, PhD

## Books & Audiobooks by Blythe Ayne

### Nonfiction:
#### How to Save Your Life Series:
Save Your Life with Awesome Apple Cider Vinegar
Save Your Life with the Dynamic Duo – D3 and K2
Save Your Life With The Power Of pH Balance
Save Your Life With The Phenomenal Lemon
Save Your Life with Basic Baking Soda
Save Your Life with Stupendous Spices
Save Your Life with the Elixir of Water

#### Absolute Beginner Series:
Chair Yoga – Easy, Healing Moves You Can Do with a Chair
Bed Yoga – Easy, Healing, Yoga Moves You Can Do in Bed
Bed Yoga for Couples—Easy, Healing, Yoga Moves You Can Do in Bed
Write Your Book! Publish Your Book! Market Your Book!

#### Excellent Life Series:
Love Is The Answer
45 Ways To Excellent Life
Horn of Plenty–The Cornucopia of Your Life
Finding Your Path, Engaging Your Purpose

### Novels:
#### Joy Forest Mysteries:
A Loveliness of Ladybugs
A Haras of Horses
A Clowder of Cats
A Gaggle of Geese

#### Women's Fiction
Eos

#### The Darling Undesirables Series:
The Heart of Leo - novelette prequel
The Darling Undesirables
Moons Rising
The Inventor's Clone
Heart's Quest

#### Middle Grade Fiction:
Matthew's Forest

#### The People in the Mirror Series:
(with Thea Thomas)
The People in the Mirror
Millie in the Mirror
The Angel in the Mirror

#### Children's Illustrated Books:
The Rat Who Didn't Like Rats
The Rat Who Didn't Like Christmas

#### Novellas & Short Story Collections:
5 Minute Stories
13 Lovely Frights for Lonely Nights
When Fields Hum & Glow

***Poetry & Photography***
*Home & the Surrounding Territory*
*Life Flows on the River of Love*
***Audiobooks:***
*Save Your Life With The Phenomenal Lemon*
*Save Your Life with Stupendous Spices*
*The Darling Undesirables*
*The Heart of Leo*
*The People in the Mirror*

*Blythe Ayne's paperback, large print, hardback books, ebooks, & audiobooks may be purchased wherever books are sold*

*and at: https://shop.BlytheAyne.com*
*www.BlytheAyne.com*

***Dedication:***

*To all who seek to live a*
*Healthier, Happier, Love-filled Life.*

# Table of Contents

# Chair Yoga

## The Great Yoga Alternative for Everyone!

### Who is Chair Yoga For?

Chair yoga is for anyone! Whether you have bodily constraints, if you're recovering from an injury, or if you're in the office and going stir crazy sitting in a chair all day. Whether you're older or younger, if you have a chair you can get a great workout using this prop.

You can enjoy your chair yoga super slow and easy, imagining the move in your mind's eye, while consciously firing the muscles involved in that move, even if you're not able to fully engage in it.

Or you can take it to another level altogether, using the chair as a prop to push further into the asanas, the moves, than you do when only on the mat.

That is to say, chair yoga is for you, no matter your level of practice. You only need to remember that even though chair yoga is for everyone, you get to decide which poses do the most for you. If you are dealing with mobility or balance issues, work with the poses that are the most beneficial for you.

Be sure to talk with a healthcare professional who clearly understands your goals, and who will work with you to reach them.

Central to everyone's yoga practice is to *always breathe deeply!* Your breath feeds your bones, ligaments, sinews, cartilage, facia, tendons, muscles, organs, joints, bursae, blood, lymph, skin … every little molecule of you!

But please do keep in mind to *never* push to a point of pain. In yoga, there's no place for the notion of "no pain, no gain." The gain in yoga is the experience of becoming familiar with the flexible and the inflexible parts of your body.

*Love them all!* Yoga is not a competition. It's so much better than any notion of competition. It's a terrain of self-learning, and self-loving, built upon the integration of mind, heart, and body.

> Yoga is the exploration
> & discovery
> Of the subtle
> Energies of Life.
> Amit Ray

## *Your Yoga Chair!*

Your special friend in chair yoga is, of course, *the chair*. It can be any armless chair – a folding chair, a lovely, flowery upholstered chair, a dining room chair, or an office chair.

It can even be a chair with arms, such as you might be limited to, say, in an airport. You can adapt accordingly. The chair is your prop to do with as best suits your needs.

The most important thing to keep in mind regarding your chair is that it is solidly situated – an advantage of fixed airport chairs! Your chair must not slide around. Place it on a yoga mat or brace it against a wall. Lock the wheels on a wheeled office chair. Just be sure, before beginning, that your chair will take your weight pushing against it without moving.

You may want to have at hand a folded blanket and a yoga block, or a few books to use as additional props for some of the poses.

So … *Let's begin!*

# Chair Yoga

# The Poses

# *Seated Head & Neck Tilt and Rolls*

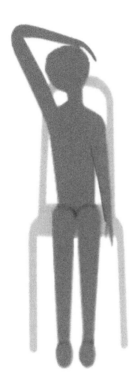

## *Movement:*

Sit in your chair feet firmly on the floor, hands in your lap, with a straight spine, ears over shoulders, shoulders over hips. If your feet do not firmly rest on the floor, use a yoga block, a folded blanket, or a couple of books under your feet to have a strong circuit of groundedness in this seated position.

Breathe deeply.

Bring your right hand over your head to your left ear, gently reaching your right ear toward your right shoulder. Hold it there for 3 to 5 deep breaths, feeling the muscles in your neck relax. Then lower your arm and raise your head.

Take your left arm and bring it over your head to your right ear, and gently bring your left ear toward your left shoulder, holding for the same amount of breaths as you did on the other side, feeling the muscles release and relax.

Return your left hand to your lap and raise your head. Breathe deeply, continuing to feel the relaxation in your neck.

Now bring your arms to your knees. Inhale and roll your head to the left, reaching the jaw bone to your shoulder, exhale, roll your head to your chest, inhale, roll to your right shoulder, reaching the jaw bone to your shoulder, then exhale, gently rolling your head back, looking up, and inhale, around to your left shoulder again.

Repeat this neck roll three or four times. Then reverse the roll in the opposite direction, the same number of times.

Think about all the demands your neck fulfills, that narrow isthmus, that communicates everything from the brain to the body, and the body to the brain. It's not hard to realize that it needs special love and attention. If all you have time for is a few neck rolls, it will be time well invested. And neck rolls can be accomplished anytime, anywhere, regardless of the chair!

**Benefits**:

Neck rolls help relieve headaches, as well as other neck, shoulder, or upper back pains. It also helps you keep the right position of your head, reducing strain on your neck. The muscles are strengthened and tension is released.

Yoga is the dance
of every cell
With the music
of every breath.

Debasish Mridha

# Cat – Marjariasana, Cow – Bitilasana

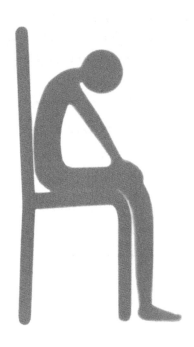

## Movement:

Now then, your spine is envious of the attention your neck got! So let's move into some spine flexing, *Cat-Cow* stretches.

With your hands on your thighs, curl your spine, chin to chest, visualizing a cat arching her back, while each vertebra gains a bit of distance from its neighbors.

Breathe deeply. The oxygen is feeding your spine, nurturing each and every vertebra. Hold this pose for a few seconds, continuing to breathe deeply, enjoying the release.

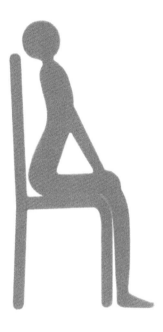

Then reverse the pose. Your vertebrae, like a string of pearls, gradually come into a forward curve, vertebrae by vertebrae. Raise your head, imagining a lovely cow looking up at the clouds passing overhead. Hold this pose for a few seconds, or as long as it feels good, while continuing to breathe deeply.

Repeat your cat-cow three to five times. Your spine says, *"Thank you!"*

## Benefits:

*Cat-Cow* stretches, strengthen, and lengthen your spine. They release tension in the neck and upper back. The cow pose nurtures your tailbone, the root of the spine.

*Cat-Cow* pose also stretches your abdomen, hips, and chest, while caring for your lungs, improving blood flow in the spine and pelvis. *Cat-Cow* poses also release tight muscles in the shoulders. Altogether they serve to increase your flexibility for all forward and backward bends and contribute to keeping the space between your vertebrae while improving the circulation of spinal fluid.

Breathing slowly and opening the chest during the cow pose helps to expand your diaphragm, contributing to the health of your heart and lungs. Awareness of your spine, and how coordinating your breath with spine movements makes you more aware of the center of your body, contributing to a straight and beautiful posture.

Its massaging effect on the abdomen aids digestion and the abdominal expansion and contraction provide healthful stimulation for your kidneys, the liver, and your thyroid gland.

*Cat-Cow* stimulates a bodily energy flow while producing a calm mind, helping to activate the parasympathetic nervous system. *Cat Pose* contributes to relieving sciatic pain.

When the entire spine is stretched, it stimulates the flow of prana, life force, from tailbone to head, energizing the brain. This is helpful for people who suffer from insomnia and migraines and provides peaceful emotional balance. *Cat-Cow* helps release anger and addictive inclinations, replacing them with focus and creativity.

May all beings have
Happy minds.
Buddha

# Seated Twist – Ardha Matsyendrasana

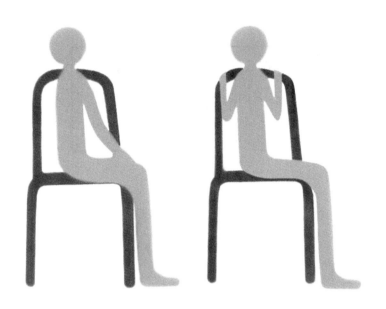

**Movement**:

Turn to the right to sit sideways in your chair, with your hands in your lap. Then twist to your right, holding onto the back of the chair. Look over your right shoulder, reaching into the twist, as far as it is comfortable. Hold this position for 5 to 10 deep breaths, or more if you are enjoying the pose.

Undo the twist, returning your hands to your lap, then repeat the twist 2 to 5 more times.

Then turn your body to the left side of the chair and twist to the left, holding on to the back of the chair. Look over your left shoulder, enjoying the twist, holding the position for the same number of deep breaths as you did on the right side. Repeat the twist the same number of times, as well.

## *Benefits*:

Twists increase spinal flexibility and help you move more freely in your body. Seated spinal twists relieve lower back pain, improve spinal flexibility, strengthen your core, massage internal organs, and promote healthy digestion.

Beyond meditation
There is the experience
Of Now.

Ryan Parenti

# Leg Lift – Anantasana

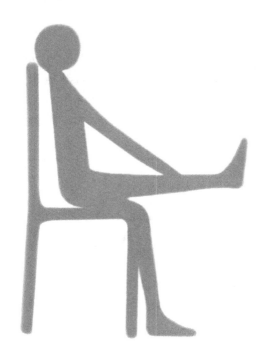

## Movement:

Sitting straight in your chair, extend your right leg out in front of you as straight as you can, holding onto your thigh with your hands for 5 to 10 deep breaths, releasing all the tension in your body and lowering your shoulders. Then release your foot back to the floor.

If you discover that you can't reach your leg straight out, lift it to where it's comfortable, keeping your back straight, and breathing deeply.

Then repeat the same process with your left leg. It's not unusual to learn that your two sides are different!

Repeat the leg lifts 2 to 3 times, or as many times as it feels comfortable.

You can also place a yoga strap or a belt around your foot, flexing your foot and straightening your leg, which may be helpful to extend your leg. Release all the tension in your body, and lower your shoulders.

### *Benefits*:

Leg lifts are a great way to get a good hamstring stretch. This pose also tones your kidneys, liver, and spleen, while improving digestion and circulation. It will also reduce swelling in the legs.

Remember to breathe.
It is, after all,
The secret to life.

Gregory Maguire

# Boat Pose – Paripurna Navasana

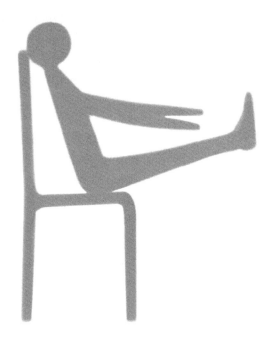

## *Movement*:

Move a bit forward on the chair and lean back. Breathe deeply. Keeping your back straight, raise both legs and reach toward them with your arms. This requires more leg strength than the leg lifts, and you may only be able to raise your two legs a short distance. Breathe deeply for 2 to 5 breaths, then relax your legs and sit up.

Repeat *Boat Pose* once again. You can also use the strap around both legs. Keep your back straight and extend into your boat pose. Conversely, you can bend your knees while raising both legs. The objective is to do the pose from where you are. Remember, *no judgment!*

### *Benefits*:

*Boat Pose* strengthens the core, hips, abdomen, and groin, and contributes to better control over your arms and legs. It opens the throat, shoulders, and chest, and lengthens the neck and spine.

It improves posture, balance, circulation, and digestion, tones your midsection, and builds up your lumbar area while improving concentration and focus.

May you pass on the Love
That has been
Given to you.
St. Terese of Lizzequx

# Seated Wide-Legged Forward Bend – Upavistha Konasana

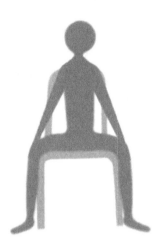

**Movement**:

Sit up straight in your chair and move your legs to the two front corners of the seat. You may need yoga blocks or books under your feet, so they can rest comfortably on a surface.

Place your hands on your thighs or your knees, whichever gives you a comfortable stretch, and slowly, *s-l-o-w-l-y* reach your torso and arms forward to touch the floor, or as far as you can comfortably reach. Breathe deeply for 5 to 10 breaths, picturing the wonderful stretch in your vertebrae, shoulders, and arms.

Come up *v-e-r-y s-l-o-w-l-y*, even more slowly than you folded forward. If you feel a bit dizzy, sit calmly with your hands in your lap, breathing deeply. Repeat the pose once or twice more.

## *Benefits*:

*Wide-Legged Forward Bend* benefits the lower back, hips, pelvis, core, glutes, quadriceps, and hamstrings while increasing muscle elasticity and strength.

As the shoulders, chest, abdomen, hips, back, and legs stretch into this pose, it produces an overall increase in flexibility and range of motion. The inversion of this pose with your head below your heart helps deoxygenated blood return to the heart, as well as benefiting the digestive and lymphatic systems.

Stiffness in the lower back, glutes, and hamstrings is released while giving the internal organs a gentle massage. The inversion can also be effective for improving sinusitis or nasal allergies, as it flushes blocked sinuses.

*Wide-Legged Forward Bend* can also help improve sciatica, back pain, and even varicose veins.

Yoga poses with the feet far apart work to improve physical and emotional stability, increasing confidence and self-control.

> Yoga is stilling the
> Changing states of mind.
> Patanjali

# *Standing Pose – Tadasana*

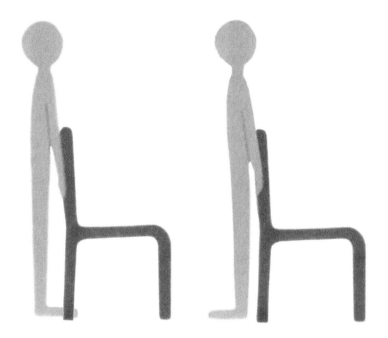

## *Movement*:

Let's do some standing poses with the chair. The classic starting point with standing poses is *Tadasana*. You may either face the back of your chair or stand with your back to the back of your chair, whichever is more comfortable.

With your ears over shoulders, shoulders over hips, and hips over knees, use the chair for support, while the ultimate goal is to stand with your hands at your sides, palms facing forward.

Hold this standing pose, breathing deeply. Imagine your breath circulating through your entire body, from the top of your head to the very ends of your fingers and toes. Hold *Tadasana* for as long as is comfortable, which may only be a few seconds, or a couple of minutes.

## *Benefits*:

*Tadasana* improves your coordination and posture. It contributes to agility, relieves sciatic pain, improves circulation, and tones your core muscles while strengthening your back, hips, and legs. Focusing on your breath and your body while quietly holding this position increases your awareness of your thoughts, promotes mental clarity, and brings you into the present moment.

The heart
Of yoga practice
Is a steady effort
In the direction
You want to go.
Sally Kempton

# Star Pose – Utthita Tadasana

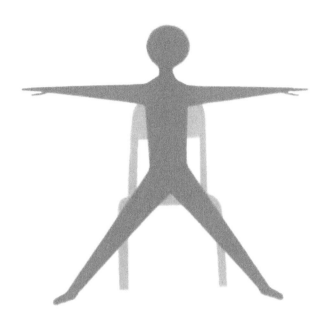

## Movement:

You may lean against your secure chair for support. Take a wide stance with your legs and reach your arms straight out from your sides with your palms facing forward, keeping your chin parallel to the floor. Have your wrists and your feet the same distance apart, with wrists over ankles, and ears, shoulders, and hips all in a line.

Feel firmly grounded through your feet, pressing all four corners of both feet evenly into the earth. Tuck your tailbone

slightly, keeping your back straight. Inhale, picturing your torso lengthening, and exhale, lowering your shoulder blades.
Expand your collarbones and extend this energy to your fingers and out through your fingertips, rotating your arms out slightly.

Energize your body with your breath in star pose, inhaling and exhaling deeply for 10 to 20 breaths, feeling your body extend in all directions with every exhale.

### *Benefits*:
*Star Pose* engages every muscle in the body, aligning the spine and strengthening your abdomen, back, legs, and ankles. It improves circulation and respiration due to providing expanded space for the heart and lungs. It improves posture, flat feet, and sciatica, and reduces back and shoulder pain.

Emotionally, *Star Pose* improves concentration and relieves stress. The open stance welcomes happiness and love.

> Feelings come and go
> Like clouds in a windy sky.
> Conscious breathing
> Is my anchor.
> Thich Nhat Hanh

# Goddess – Utkata Konasana

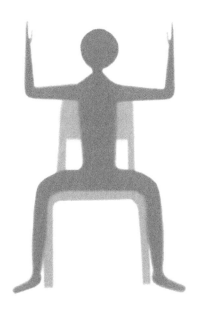

***Movement:***

You can do *Goddess Pose* standing or sitting. The following instructions are for the seated position. Move your legs to the corners of your chair so that your knees are pointed in opposite directions, and add energy to your pose by pressing your knees toward the back of the chair. Maintain a straight spine. Breathing deeply, raise your hands into a cactus position.

To progress with your *Goddess Pose*, bring yourself to standing, bend your knees, and come down to the chair, just shy of sitting. Don't forget to breathe!

An excellent flow is from *Star Pose* to *Goddess Pose*. Try cycling through the two poses several times, and see how energizing this flow feels!

## *Benefits*:

*Goddess Pose* is a powerful stretch for your hips, glutes, adductors, pelvic floor, psoas, quadriceps, knees, ankles, and feet. Cactus arms strengthen your neck, shoulders, upper back, chest, rib cage, diaphragm, breathing muscles, and arms, bringing about deeper breathing and improved lung capacity.

The intensity of this pose requires concentration and focus. It counteracts the damage of sitting at a desk for hours, increasing blood circulation at the pelvic floor. The flow of prana, which is energy, flushes out stagnant energy, and brings in fresh energy. This flow of energy stimulates the organs while calming the nervous system.

The result is elevated confidence and self-esteem while setting aside negative emotions. *Goddess Pose* brings harmony to your physical, mental, emotional, and spiritual bodies.

Move the way
Love makes you move.
Osho

# Downward Facing Dog –
## Adho Mukha Svanasana

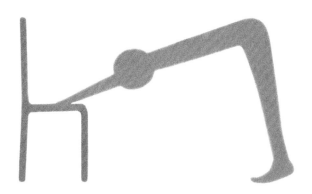

## *Movement*:

Face the front of your chair. Making sure that the chair is secure, place your hands on the seat of the chair, and step your feet back so that you make an upside-down V with your spine and legs. Gradually reach your heels to touch the floor.

A modification is to not reach quite so far back with your legs and feet, and bend your knees. A straight spine is the primary objective of *Downward-Facing Dog*. Hold your *Downward-Facing Dog* for 10 to 15 deep breaths.

## *Benefits*:

*Downward-Facing Dog* increases blood flow to the head, which, *bonus!*, supplies nutrients to your hair, improves hearing, and eyesight, and stimulates a glowing complexion. The blood flow to your brain improves memory while reducing anxiety, depression, and panic attacks. You may also discover it banishes insomnia. It will quell digestion problems, gas, and acidity.

It is also helpful in improving constipation and varicose veins. It strengthens the core and tones hands and legs, while increasing flexibility, strengthening you from your neck and shoulders all the way to your hamstrings and calves.

> Yoga is the addition
> of energy, strength
> & beauty
> To body, mind & soul.
>
> Amit Ray

# Upward-Facing Dog –
# Urdhva Mukha Svanasana

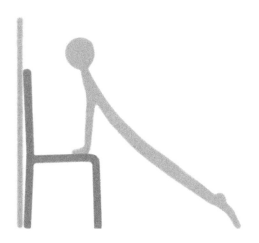

## *Movement*:

For *Upward-Facing Dog*, you must make doubly certain the chair is secure, preferably against the wall. Breathing deeply, press firmly downward with your hands, *not your wrists!* on the seat of the chair, and walk your feet back until you are in a plank position, with your back and legs nearly straight.

Press your hips and torso forward. Keep your shoulders down from your ears, and your legs lifted. This pose requires quite a bit of strength, so be patient with yourself while practicing it. *Don't overdo!*

You will notice that you can flow from *Downward-Facing Dog* to *Upward-Facing Dog*.

**Benefits**:
*Upward-Facing Dog* is a deep backbend, which powerfully strengthens your core, as well as building up your wrists, arms, and back.

It's the perfect answer to hunkering over a desk all day with its chest-opening action. At the same time, it opens the heart and the lungs and improves digestion. This opening provides an emotional component as well, reducing feelings of depression or overwhelm.

Liberate yourself
From your fears
& your presence liberates
Others from theirs.

Marianne Williamson

# Lunge – Utthita Ashwa Sanchalanasana

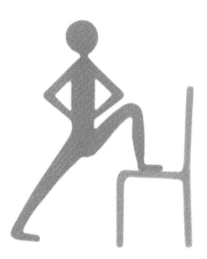

*Movement*:

Step back from the front of the chair. Reach forward to hold on to the back of the chair, then raise your right foot onto the seat of the chair while reaching your left leg behind you into an extended, comfortable stretch. Removing your hands, raise your torso perpendicular to the floor. Square your hips so that they both face forward.

Straightening and bending the right leg may help you settle into the pose. Place your hands on your thighs or on your hips, whichever is more comfortable.

Enjoy the pose, breathing deeply for 5 to 10 breaths.

Then repeat the *Lunge* with your left foot on the seat of the chair, your hands on the back of the chair for support, and reaching the right foot back into an extended stretch. Removing your hands, raise your torso perpendicular to the floor.

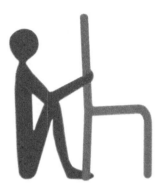

Again, square your hips so they face forward.

Straighten and bend the left knee to help settle into the pose. Place your hands on your thighs or on your hips, whichever is more comfortable.

Breathe deeply for 5 to 10 breaths.

### *Benefits*:
*Lunge* increases strength and stamina in your arms, back, knees, hips, quadriceps, glutes, hamstrings, and calf muscles. It stretches the psoas muscles, engages core muscles, alleviates sciatic pain, improves balance, and helps you get into the habit of squaring your hips.

> Yoga teaches us to
> Cure what need not
> Be endured
> & endure what cannot
> Be cured.
>
> B.K.S. Iyengar

# Squat – Garland Pose – Malasana

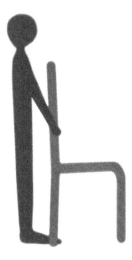

## Movement:

Hold on to the back of your chair with your feet hips width apart and your pelvis slightly tilted forward. Engage your core, and inhale deeply.

Exhale and bend your knees, *slowly* squatting down. Continue to breathe deeply as you slowly reach your hips down and back as though you are about to sit on the edge of a chair, but continue down as far as you can go. Bring your weight to the heels of your feet. If your heels do not reach the floor, have a folded blanket within reach to put under your heels.

After several deep breaths, engage your glutes and push into your thighs and feet to return to standing.

*A full Garland Pose is not easy!* You may not be able to go very far down. Take it as far as you can safely go without abusing your knees. Over time, you'll be pleased to discover that you're able to go farther down into your squat. One of the best pay-offs for working on your squat is building up the strength in your knees.

Be patient, and be persevering.

## *Benefits*:
*Garland Pose* stretches and strengthens your muscles, joints, ankles, groin, and back while stimulating digestion. It facilitates the health and strength of your pelvic floor. It opens your hips, and groin, which reduces low back pain, eliminates toxins, and gets the digestive system in great working order.

It is also a powerful means of correcting and improving your posture due to the spinal alignment and balance in the hips.

*Garland Pose* makes you feel more grounded, bringing you down to earth and calming you. It's a great preparation for meditation or a good night's sleep.

Yoga traditions believe that stress and negative emotions are stored in the hips. *Garland Pose* helps you release these counterproductive emotions. As it is centered on the sacral chakra, it opens up the flow of creativity.

Once you understand
The grammar of yoga
You can write
Your poetry of movement.
Amit Ray

# Lord of the Dance – Natarajasana

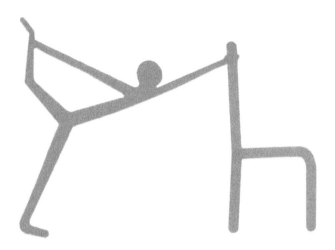

## *Movement*:

Place a chair in front of you with its back to you. Breathing deeply, stand straight, then place your right hand on the top of the chair for support. Lift your left foot behind you, and reach back with your left hand to hold onto the inside of your left foot. Press your right thigh into your hip joint and raise your kneecap for stability.

Holding your left foot, stretch your left side until it's parallel to the floor. Hold the pose for several breaths, then return your foot to the floor, standing straight.

Repeat the pose on the opposite side, breathing deeply, placing your left hand on the chair for support and lifting your right foot behind you, reaching it with your right hand, and holding onto the inside of your foot.

Without the chair, this is considered an advanced move. Work with the pose in small increments, and you will see your flexibility improve.

### *Benefits*:

*Lord of the Dance* is named after the Hindu god, Shiva Nataraja, often seen in a dancing pose. This pose builds your ankles and legs, while simultaneously stretching your chest, shoulders, abdomen, thighs, and groin, all of which help to improve balance.

*Lord of the Dance* opens your shoulders and chest, increases lung capacity, strengthens leg muscles and the arches of your feet, and tones your spine.

It helps develop poise, and emotionally it energizes your mind, reduces stress, anxiety, and depression.

Quiet the mind
& the Soul will speak.
Anonymous

# Chair Pose – Utkatasana

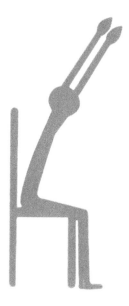

## *Movement*:

Chair pose is *Utkatasana* in Sanskrit, which means "powerful, wild, or fierce pose." This pose is not as easy as it looks. It's a challenging standing pose that tests different parts of your body.

*Let's try it!*

Standing with your arms outstretched overhead, bend your knees, lowering to your chair, but hover just shy of sitting. Breathe deeply and hold this position. If you cannot hold it, become seated while maintaining the sensation of engaged muscles in the legs and back. Employ this pose gently if you have knee or ankle issues.

Keep working with this pose until you can hover over your chair for several seconds, adding strength to your thighs, lower back, and torso.

If you *can* hover in the air-seated position, the challenge is to lengthen the amount of time you can hold your fierce pose.

### *Benefits*:
Chair pose builds strength in your spine, hips, and chest, and tones your thighs, knees, and ankle muscles.

It improves balance, while at the same time, it has the emotional component of nurturing determination and fulfilling goals.

> Practice gratitude
> While practicing yoga.
> Blythe Ayne

# *Push-up – Chaturanga*

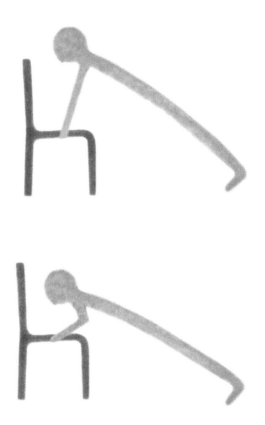

## *Movement*:

Making sure your chair is very secure, place your hands on the edge of the seat, with your hands, elbows, and shoulders in a straight line. Engage your core and step back into a plank pose, with your back and legs long and straight.

Breathing deeply, keeping your elbows close to your body, slowly lower your elbows moving your torso toward the chair. Then straighten your arms again.

If this pose is a challenge, lower your elbows only a couple of inches then straighten your arms. Do this three times.

If this pose is relatively easy for you, the challenge is to add repetitions.

Chaturanga requires a lot of strength, and if you're not ready for it, you can save it for later Remember, this is *your* yoga practice, and you decide which poses you're ready to engage in!

## *Benefits*:
Yoga push-ups strengthen and tone your wrists, arms, lower back, the muscles surrounding your spine, and abdominal muscles, improving core strength and core stability, and contributing to aligning your whole body.

Chaturanga boosts confidence and helps balance emotions.

Letting go
Is the hardest asana.

Anonymous

# Wide-Legged Forward Fold – Prasarita Padottanasana

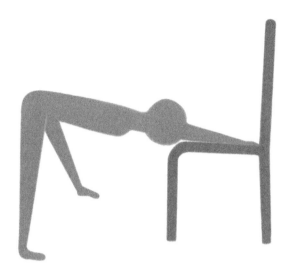

## *Movement*:

Standing in front of your chair, take a wide-legged stance and reach forward to the seat of the chair. Breathing deeply, rest your arms on the seat of the chair, while maintaining a straight line from your hands to your hips, and engaging the muscles in your legs. Keep your shoulder blades drawn together and down your back and keep the front of your body open. Breathe deeply for 5 to 10 breaths before returning to a standing position.

***Benefits***:

*Wide-Legged Forward Fold* is a great stretch for your hamstrings, back, and the insides of your thighs. It opens the hips and stretches the spine, shoulders, and chest while easing tension in the upper back. It counteracts the effects of sitting at a desk all day.

Inversions also bathe the brain with freshly oxygenated blood, with all of the benefits that that implies, including calming and relaxing the mind from anxious feelings and thoughts, while easing tension headaches.

> The more you see
> The good in others
> The more you see
> The good in yourself.
> Pramahansa Yogananda

# *Tree – Vrksasana*

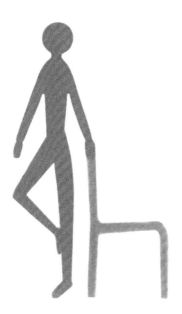

## *Movement*:

Hold on to the back of your chair with your left hand. Breathing deeply and feeling grounded with your left foot, raise your right foot to rest against your left ankle.

If you would like to go a bit further in this balancing pose, you can raise your right foot and rest it on your left calf. If you are yet more flexible, you can raise your right foot to your inner thigh. Avoid resting your foot against your precious knee. It needs to hold you up for at least 100 years!

You can continue to hold on to the chair for balance with your left hand while extending your right hand out to the side, or overhead like branches, or together in front of your heart in prayer pose.

If adventuresome, see if you can remove your left hand to mirror your right hand, in a full balancing pose.

Even if you only hold this pose for a few seconds, that's fantastic! You'll get better as you continue your tree practice.

When you have completed tree on this side, turn and hold on to the back of your chair with your right hand, feeling grounded down into your roots with your right foot, and raising your left foot to rest against your ankle, your calf, or your thigh, breathing deeply.

Continue to hold on to the chair for balance with your right hand, or practice your balance by letting it join the poses of your left hand.

When completed, return your left foot to the floor with your hands in prayer position before your heart, sending up a little prayer of gratitude for your amazing body.

### *Benefits*:
*Tree Pose* is a balancing and grounding pose that strengthens your bones, spine, glutes, thighs, calves, and ankles, and stretches the shoulders, chest, groin, and thighs. It improves posture after sitting for hours.

It opens the energy centers along the spine, helps with focus and concentration, while at the same time, it balances and energizes your chakras.

> The health of your mind
> Depends on
> Your being able to
> Love your body.
>
> Rodney Yee

# Warrior One – Verabhadrasana

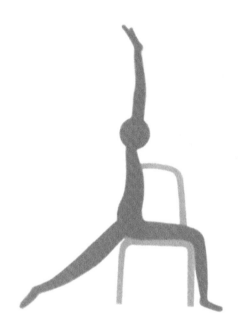

## *Movement*:

With the back of your chair to your right, move to the edge of the chair, and extend your left leg behind, with your foot at a 45-degree angle, and firmly grounded. Your right thigh is across the seat of the chair, with your knee bent at a 90-degree angle and touching the floor. If it does not touch the floor, support it with a yoga block or books. The right and left heels should be in a line.

Inhaling deeply, reach your arms up overhead, with palms facing each other, shoulder blades open out, away from your spine. Then rotate your biceps back while firming your triceps. Keep your gaze forward, and breathe deeply, holding the pose for 5 to 10 breaths.

Release the pose, and repeat on the opposite side, with the back of your chair to your left, extend your right leg behind with your foot at a 45-degree angle, firmly grounded. Your left thigh is across the seat of the chair, with your knee bent at a 90-degree angle, touching the floor, or your yoga block, or books. The left and right heels are in a line.

Inhale deeply, reach your arms overhead, palms facing, shoulder blades open, away from your spine. Rotate your biceps, firming your triceps. Keep your drishti, that is, your gaze, forward, breathing deeply, holding the pose for the same number of breaths as on the other side.

## *Benefits*:
*Warrior Poses* build stamina, and improve coordination. *Warrior I* strengthens your core, glutes, hip flexors, shins, and feet. It also strengthens the upper body, stretching your torso from the psoas up to your shoulders. It also strengthens the shoulders and arms, improving posture and undoing the negative effects of hours of computer work.

The beauty of *Warrior I* is that it engages balancing simultaneous movements in different directions to manifest stillness. The result is a sense of profound potential energy.

Go from a human being
Doing yoga
To a human
Being yoga.

Baron Baptiste

# Warrior II – Verabhadrasana II

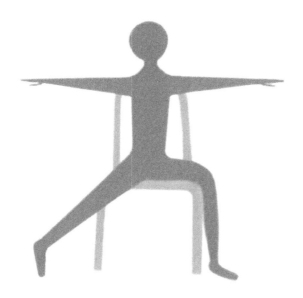

**Movement:**

The core movements of *Warrior II* are essentially the same as *Warrior I.* With the back of your chair to your right, move to the edge of the chair, and extend your left leg behind, with your foot at a 45-degree angle, and firmly grounded. Your right thigh is across the seat of the chair, with your knee bent at a 90-degree angle and touching the floor. If it does not touch the floor, support it with a yoga block or books. The right and left heels should be in a line.

Lift your arms parallel to the floor, turn your palms and inner elbows to face the ceiling, drawing your shoulder blades down your back. Keeping your shoulder blades extended down, turn your palms to face down again.

Keep your head and shoulders centered over your hips. Extend energy through your arms and gaze beyond the fingertips of your right hand, breathing deeply for 5 to 10 breaths. Exhale and relax the pose.

Then move to the other side, and repeat, moving so that the back of your chair is to your left. Extend your right leg behind, with your foot at a 45-degree angle, and firmly grounded. Your left thigh is across the seat of the chair, with your knee bent at a 90-degree angle and touching the floor. If it does not touch the floor, support it with a yoga block or books. The left and right heels should be in a line.

Lift your arms parallel to the floor, turn your palms and inner elbows to face the ceiling, drawing your shoulder blades down your back. Keeping your shoulder blades extended down, turn your palms to face down again.

Keep your head and shoulders centered over your hips. Extend energy through your arms, and gaze beyond the fingertips of your left hand, breathing deeply for 5 to 10 breaths. Exhale and relax the pose.

### *Benefits*:
*Warrior II* strengthens your core, your back muscles, hip flexors, gluteal muscles, inner thigh, hamstrings, calf muscles, and an-

kles. It stretches and strengthens your shoulders and chest, increasing endurance. It improves posture and is grounding, opening, and lengthening, a powerful combination.

All these attributes have the effect of strengthening your focus and resolve.

> The pose begins
> When you want to
> Get out of it.
>
> Baron Baptiste

# Reverse Warrior – Viparita Virabhadrasana

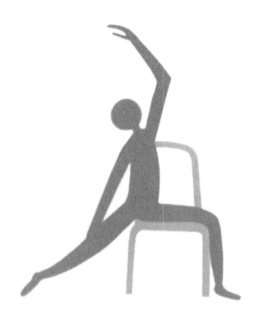

## Movement:

*Reverse Warrior* is, once again, the same essential setup and pose as the previous warrior poses. With the back of your chair to your right, move to the edge of the chair, and extend your left leg behind, with your foot at a 45-degree angle, and firmly grounded. Your right thigh is across the seat of the chair, with your knee bent at a 90-degree angle and touching the floor. If it does not touch the floor, support it with a yoga block or books. The right and left heels should be in a line.

Bring your left arm to the left leg and lift the right arm toward the ceiling on an exhale.

Keep your head and shoulders centered over your hips. Breathing deeply, extend energy through your arms, and lift your gaze to your raised hand, breathing deeply for 5 to 10 breaths. Exhale and relax the pose.

Then move to the other side, and repeat, moving so that the back of your chair is to your left. Extend your right leg behind, with your foot at a 45-degree angle, and firmly grounded. Your left thigh is across the seat of the chair, with your knee bent at a 90-degree angle and touching the floor. If it does not touch the floor, support it with a yoga block or books. The left and right heels should be in a line.

Bring your left arm to the left leg and lift the right arm toward the ceiling on an exhale.

Keep your head and shoulders centered over your hips. Breathing deeply, extend energy through your arms, and lift your gaze to your raised hand, breathing deeply for 5 to 10 breaths. Exhale and relax the pose.

### *Benefits*:

Like *Warrior II, Reverse Warrior* strengthens your core, your back muscles, hip flexors, gluteal muscles, inner thigh, hamstrings, calf muscles, and ankles. It stretches and strengthens your shoulders and chest, increasing endurance. It is grounding and improves posture. It is opening, and lengthening, a powerful combination.

All these attributes have the effect of strengthening your focus and resolve.

> The most important
> Moment in a day
> Is the rest we take
> Between two deep breaths.
> Etty Hillesum

# Half Pigeon – Ardha Kapotasana

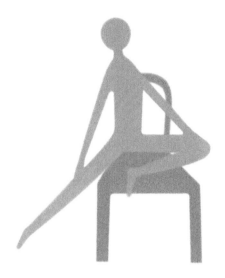

## *Movement*:

Sitting to the left back and diagonally on your chair, breathe deeply and gently bend your right knee, bringing your leg onto the front of the chair. Move your left leg behind you and touch the floor with your toes pointed, or place your foot facing down if it is comfortable to do so.

Reach your arms to your thighs, and breathe deeply for 5 to 10 breaths into the pose.

To take *Half Pigeon* to the next level, bring your hands to your right thigh and shin, and bend over your right thigh.

Then repeat the pose on the other side.
Sit to the right back and diagonally on your chair, breathe deeply, and gently bend your left knee, bringing your leg onto the front of the chair. Move your right leg behind you and touch the floor with your toes pointed, or place your foot facing down if it is comfortable to do so.

Reach your arms to your thighs, and breathe deeply for 5 to 10 breaths into the pose.

If you would like to take the pose to the next level, bring your hands to your left thigh and shin and bend over your left thigh.

### *Benefits*:
*Half Pigeon* deeply opens the hips. It cleanses the liver and produces restorative energy. It lengthens the hip flexors and increases the range of motion of the femur. It increases the outward rotation of the femur in the hip socket, while lengthening the psoas muscle, connecting the torso and the legs. This muscle can become chronically, and most painfully, shortened in our chair-bound society.

It is a pose that gently releases stored negative emotions, and clears them out.

To conquer the unknown
You must trust.

Yogi Bhagan

# *Butterfly – Supta Baddha Konasana*

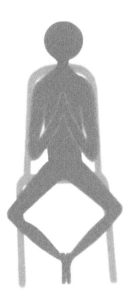

## *Movement*:

Sit close to the outer edge of your chair. Make sure you feel comfortable and stable. Breathe deeply and touch the soles of your feet to the floor, then bring them together to face each other, letting your knees fall out to the sides. If your feet do not touch the floor you can place a block or books under them. Root down into your sitting bones and legs.

Tuck your chin to your chest while elongating and straightening your spine. Inhale and lengthen your spine, feeling the energy from your toes and extending up through the top of your head. With each exhale, relax into the stretch. Hold your butterfly pose for up to two minutes.

## **Benefits**:

*Butterfly Pose* is beneficial for the muscles of your lower back, pelvic floor, hips, knees, hamstrings, ankles, and feet. It improves knee and ankle flexibility while toning the hamstrings and calf muscles.

It stimulates ovaries and prostate glands, adrenal glands, kidneys, and liver. It also stimulates the bladder meridian and the gallbladder meridian. Further, it helps relieve sciatica.

You can do *Butterfly Pose* after a meal, as it stimulates digestion.

> Yoga shines the
> Light of awareness
> Into the darkest corners
> Of the body.
> Jason Crandell

## *Open Heart*

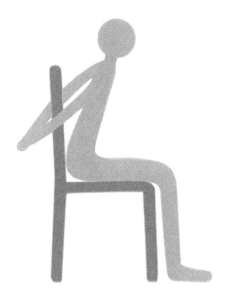

### *Movement*:

Sitting comfortably in your chair with your back straight and feet on the floor, reach your arms behind the back of the chair with your shoulder blades reaching toward each other. While breathing deeply, imagine this pose opening your heart to receive health and happiness.

If your flexibility and the back of the chair allow, clasp your hands together, extending yet further into the pose. Continue to breathe deeply, holding the pose, for a minute or two. You should not feel a strain in your shoulders, and as you come further into the pose, your shoulders will relax further.

## *Benefits*:

A heart opener pose expands the rib cage, increasing the expansion and contraction of the lungs, and thus, improving breathing. This pose also helps improve posture and reduce back pain and shoulder pain.

*Open Heart* also reduces depression, providing a burst of energy that improves your mood, and inspires motivation. It can help you heal from grief and trauma, and move you into a more positive emotional terrain.

> Bury your mind
> Deep in your heart
> & watch the body
> Move by itself.
> Sri Dharma Mittra

# Shoulder Stretch

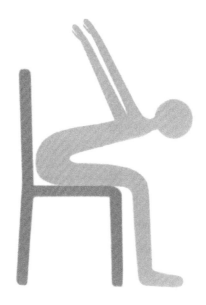

## *Movement*:

On an exhalation, fold forward from the hip joints, keeping your torso open. With your arms outstretched behind you, interlace your fingers. Breathing deeply, squeeze your elbows and shoulder blades toward each other and press your knuckles toward the ceiling while arching your back. Breathe slowly for 5 to 10 breaths, and then slowly release out of the stretch, returning your hands to your lap.

A shoulder stretch with hands clasped behind your back releases tension in the deltoids and trapezius.

## *Benefits*:

Clasping your hands behind your back releases tension in your deltoids and trapezius. Sitting at a desk typing all day causes the shoulders to slump, which leads to tightness in the neck, shoulders, and chest. A shoulder stretch is the perfect way to release that desk-computer-typing tension.

> The body benefits
> From movement
> & the mind benefits
> From stillness.
> Sakyong Mipham

# Extended Side Angle –
# Utthita Parsvakonasana

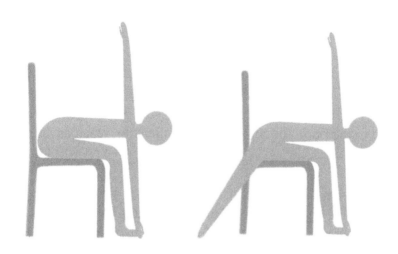

## Movement:

Sit comfortably in your chair facing forward with your feet side by side, or extend your left foot back behind the chair.

Slowly lean forward, breathing deeply and reaching your right hand to the floor. If you cannot reach the floor, reach as far as you can. Then extend your left arm straight up over-head, so that your arms are in a straight line perpendicular to the floor. Your gaze is to the left, or you can look down at your feet.

Hold the pose for 5 to 10 breaths, elongating the pose on your inhale, and going deeper into the pose with each exhale.

Come out of the pose and sit for a moment with your hands in your lap, and then repeat the pose on the left side.

Sit comfortably in your chair facing forward with your feet side by side, or extend your right foot back behind the chair. Slowly lean forward, breathing deeply and reaching your left hand to the floor. If you cannot reach the floor, reach as far as you can.

Extend your right arm up overhead, with your arms in a straight line perpendicular to the floor. Your gaze is to the left or down at your feet. Hold this pose for 5 to 10 breaths, elongating the pose on your inhale, and going deeper into the pose with each exhale.

### *Benefits*:

This is a great pose after sitting for several hours. The muscles in your sides get tight from sitting, which pulls your torso forward into a rounded position. Stretching each side of the body with an *Extended Side-Angle Pose* helps bring the body into a strong upright posture, increasing the flexibility of your joints.

It is an excellent opener of your chest and shoulders. The outstretched arms expand the muscles of the shoulders and chest, improving your breathing and giving your entire body a shot of quick energy. It tones the whole body, building strength and stamina.

*Extended Side Angle* also reduces backache and reduces sciatica, while making the spine more flexible.

Yoga.
Because punching people
Is frowned upon.

Anonymous

# Moon Salutation – Chandra Namaskara

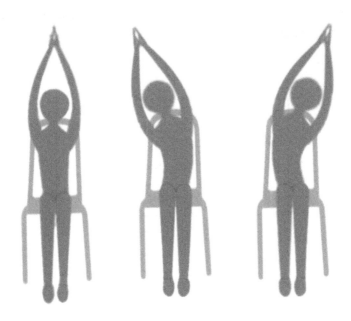

## *Movement*:

Sitting comfortably on your chair with your feet firmly plant-
ed on the floor, on an inhale, reach your arms up toward the
sky, interlacing your fingers.

On your next exhale, bend to the right, reaching as far as you
can comfortably go. Pause here for 2 to 5 breaths. On an inhale, raise your arms upward again.

On your exhale, bend to the left, reaching as far as you can
comfortably go. Pause and take the same number of breaths as

on the other side, then inhale and raise your arms overhead again.

## *Benefits*:

*Moon Salutation* strengthens the muscles of your side body, your abdomen, and your arms. It increases the function of the respiratory system and your lung capacity, while improving the alignment of your spinal column, and releasing tension in your arms, neck, and shoulders.

It helps calm the body, relieving stress and anxiety, and balances your chakras. It can improve your concentration and help you get a good night's sleep.

Yoga poses
are useful maps
To explore yourself
But they are not
The territory.
Donna Farhi

# *Easy Pose – Sukhasana*

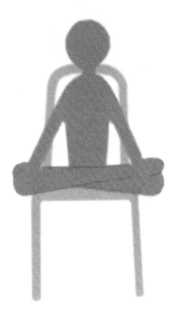

## *Movement*:

Sitting on your chair, bend your knees so that your lower legs come up on the chair, then cross your shins, with each foot underneath the opposite knee. Keep your pelvis neutral, without tilting forward or back.

Lengthen your tailbone down and pull your shoulder blades flat against your back, while lengthening your torso. Place your hands in your lap, palms up, or on your knees, palms down.

You might want to put your blanket on the chair before engaging in *Easy Pose* if it is not upholstered.

Conversely, if you cannot bring both legs to the chair, bring one leg at a time, with several breaths for each. If neither foot is flexible enough yet to come onto the chair, sit with both feet flat on the floor or your yoga block, keeping the pelvis neutral, lengthening your tailbone down, and pulling your shoulder blades flat against your back while lengthening your torso. Place your hands in your lap, palms up, or on your knees, palms down.

## *Benefits*:
*Easy Pose* is calming and relaxing if you can sit in it comfortably. It improves posture and creates a foundation for meditation.

It helps manage stress by activating the parasympathetic nervous system and deactivating the sympathetic nervous system, and helps to regulate blood pressure. Holding *Easy Pose* strengthens abdominal and spine core muscles, and stretches your groin and adductors.

Resolutely train yourself
To attain peace.
Buddha

# Bridge – Setu Bandha Sarvangasana

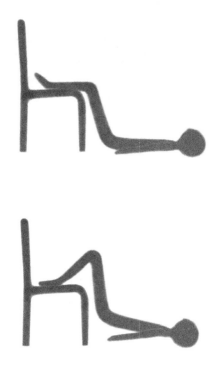

### Movement:

Let's move from the chair to the floor. Lie on your back with your knees bent at a 90-degree angle, your calves and feet on the chair.

Bring your arms alongside your body, palms down. Inhale deeply.

Pressing down firmly through your feet, lift your hips via your pubic bone, not your navel.

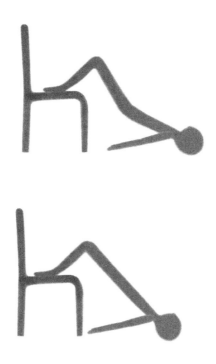

Take 3 to 5 breaths in your raised bridge, then slowly, vertebrae by vertebrae, lower your bridge, relaxing your calves on the seat of the chair.

Repeat *Bridge Pose* two or three more times. There is a tendency to hold the breath while the bridge is up – be sure to continue to breathe deeply. Keep your gaze to the ceiling, and do not turn your head while in this pose.

**Benefits**:

*Bridge Pose* gently stretches your chest, shoulders, and abdomen, strengthening your back muscles, glutes, thighs, and ankles.

It relieves low back pain and improves posture, counteracting the effects of sitting and slouching.

Because *Bridge Pose* brings your head beneath your heart, it has the many benefits of inversions, including alleviating depression and augmenting peace and joy.

Yoga not only makes
Your Body happy
It makes your
Being happy.

Blythe Ayne

# Resting Pose – Shavasana

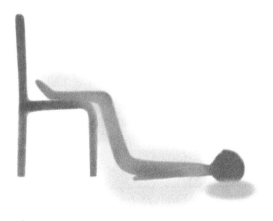

## Movement:

And now, let's assimilate our yoga practice and relax.

Lie flat on your back with your calves on the chair, and your arms at your sides. Breathe deeply. Visualize oxygen being carried to every molecule and synapse of your body.

Here, in tranquil focus, breathing deeply, enjoy affirmations of sending and receiving love. Picture a particular heart's desire becoming manifest. Meditate with equanimity, while imagining calmly sailing through even moments of challenge.

Picture yourself pausing to appreciate a flower, drinking in a work of art, stopping to listen to bird-song, and smiling warmly at others you encounter.

*What a great LIFE!*

If it's close to bedtime, picture a deep and healing sleep, affirming that you will rest peacefully and heal fully.

*Good Night! Sleep Tight!*

After giving attention to your affirmations, release it all. Let it go. Become mindful of your breathing. Breathe deeply, inhaling and exhaling—stomach rising and falling. It's good to be mindful of total, deep, breathing.

Let everything go, relaxing. *Relax.*

There is nothing to worry about. There's nothing to do. Feel your mind relaxing. Your face relaxes. Your arms and your hands ... relax. Your chest and your abdomen ... relax. Your legs and your feet ... relax. *You completely ... relax ....*

**Benefits**:
The essence of *Shavasana* is to relax with attention ... to remain conscious and alert while at ease. Remaining aware while relaxing can help you begin to notice and release long-held tensions in your body and mind.

*Shavasana* is a practice of gradually relaxing one body part at a time, one muscle at a time, one thought at a time. When you do this practice day after day, it conditions the body to release stress. It can also improve your sense of physical and emotional well-being.

But when tightness and tension have built up in your body, relaxing—even when you lie down—sometimes feels impossible. That's why it's important to practice the other, active asanas before coming to *Shavasana* because those poses stretch, open, and release tension. They also help relax the diaphragm, so the breath can move freely.

There is no difference
Between your breathing
& the breathing
Of the rain forest.
Deepak Chopra

Yoga And ....

Forms of Yoga

Pranayama ~ Yoga Breathing

Your Yoga Routines

# Yoga And ....

## Yoga Increases Range of Motion
Stiff joints and arthritic joints love a bit of yoga. Yoga is never about pushing until it hurts. In your yoga practice, you'll learn the points at which joints hurt. It's good to become conscious of the comfortable range of motion of a painful joint. We may be aware that a particular joint is painful, but not aware of the range of motion it has before it becomes painful, and so you may unknowingly push the joint beyond its optimum comfort zone.

When you learn how far the joint is comfortably flexible, you become conscious of not pushing it. With this gentle, conscious awareness, you will become successful in expanding the comfortable range of motion for that joint because of your awareness of its pain threshold.

Gentle yoga is an excellent way to slowly and mindfully increase a delicate joint's range of motion.

## Yoga Increases Muscle Strength
Also, holding poses, again, not to a point of pain, over time increases muscle strength. And muscles are the support system for joints, so in building up the muscle of a joint slowly, over time, you may discover contributes to alleviating pain.

## Yoga Builds Bones

Your bone density will also increase with a regular yoga practice. This fends off osteoporosis, or helps alleviate it, as you move toward bone strength rather than weakness.

## Yoga Banishs Anxiety & Stress

Movement relieves tension, and physical relief of tension contributes to emotional release of the tension of anxiety and stress. Mindful breathing exercises also provide relaxation and calmness in mind and body.

## Yoga & Your Lymph System

The lymph system is the powerful circulatory system of your immune system. It provides protection for our internal physiology from the daily onslaughts of toxins, bacteria, and other infections. It is largely underrated, although it's twice the size of the blood circulation system, and circulates twice the volume of blood every single day!

Western medicine, curiously, does not attend to the lymphatic system nearly as much as it should. India's *Ayurvedic* medicine is far ahead of Western medicine in this regard, considering the lymphatic system to be "the water of life."

Yoga is a great way to contribute to your healthy lymphatic system, whose job it is to clear toxins from the body. Lymphatics transport waste and toxins out of the body's tissues, to be properly disposed of. It monitors the immune system and responds to signals to increase or decrease healing inflammation, helping to protect the body against bacteria, infections, and cancer.

There are between six and eight hundred lymph nodes throughout the body, which trap pathogens, helping the immune system defend against invasion. Nodes are situated around joints, which are stimulated by pressure due to movement, and which facilitate the flow of lymphatic fluid through the nodes providing immune cells.

As the lymphatic system does not have a heart to pump it around like blood does, it is dependent on movement and pressure at joints to stimulate its flow. Yoga is fantastic support for the lymph system as both movement of joints and deep breathing act as pumps to keep the lymph in motion. Deep diaphragmatic breathing pumps the deeper lymphatics. Yoga also helps reduce stress which interferes with your body's immune response.

Another powerful component of yoga and the lymph system is inversions, such as bridge and downward dog, with your head below your heart, assisting the flow of lymph to extremities, and twists, which can be helpful wringing out nodes, and moving the lymph fluid on.

When your body is fighting an infection, the lymph nodes create more white blood cells, which causes the nodes to swell and become sensitive. This is your lymph system at work, clearing out the toxic invasion.

During your yoga practice, you might occasionally visualize your movement and breathing engaged in stimulating the lymph around your joints, and picture the lymph flowing energetically with each diaphragmatic breath, keeping you in glowing health!

Find the Peace
Within yourself
& you will live at Peace
With others.

Peace Pilgrim

## Forms of Yoga

There are many forms of yoga, each with their own emphasis. But there are two processes to keep in mind, no matter what form you engage in:

*Stay focused on your breath*—inhale and exhale through your nose to maintain your body's warmth and energy.

*Visualize your spine*—picture a comfortable space between each vertebra and disk. See, in your mind's eye, each vertebra, each disk, flexible in movement and in stillness, in perfect alignment, balanced and whole.

Many of us have vertebrae or disks that are *not* in perfect alignment, that are *not* perfectly whole, but keeping that image in your mind's eye—which is a powerful source of healing, behind *your third eye!*—can contribute to your body's ability to maintain, and to heal.

Following is a short list of the more common forms of yoga:

**Hatha Yoga** is best for the beginner as it uses a variety of common poses. It's a classic approach to yoga poses and breathing exercises.

**Iyengar Yoga** was founded by B. K. S. Iyengar. It focuses on precise movements, and the details of alignment. Poses are generally held for a long period while continuing to adjust the fine details of the pose.

*Ashtanga Yoga* the "Eight Limb path," is a physically demanding sequence of postures, generally more appropriate for the experienced yogi.

*Vinyasa Yoga* comes from *Ashtanga* as a flowing link of movements, united to the breath. It's not uncommon for a *Vinyasa* flow to be included in *Hatha* Yoga.

*Restorative Yoga* relaxes you, and, as its name implies, it restores you, body, mind, and spirit. In this relaxation and restoration, there is also rejuvenation.

No matter what time of day you engage in *Restorative Yoga*, you'll reap the benefit of the three *R's*:

*Relaxation*
*Restoration*
*Rejuvenation*

> The attitude
> Of gratitude
> Is the highest yoga.
> Yogi Bhajan

# *Pranayama – Yoga Breathing*

What if you had to consciously breathe, telling your body to do everything it requires to take a breath?

Your body is *such a miracle!* Breathing, breathing, breathing, without having to give it a moment's thought. So those times when you *do* consciously think about your breath, send gratitude to your body for breathing without being instructed.

Breathing is the most natural thing our bodies do, generously providing the fuel of life-sustaining oxygen. Breathing relieves tension and stress, calms the nervous system, and diminishes fatigue, stress, and high blood pressure with every inhale. It carts off carbon dioxide and toxins with every exhale. All are accomplished automatically.

However, central to yoga practice is *conscious attention to your breath*, altering it so that it activates your parasympathetic nervous system, the "rest and digest" system—the opposite of "fight or flight," where our harried lives hurl us far too often.

"*Prana*" is your *Life Force,* regulated by your breath. When we breathe consciously, it takes us into a grounded and meditative state. There are a number of breathing exercises in yoga. Let's consider three of the most common ones: *Ujjayi, Nadi Shodhana*, and *Kapalabhati*.

## Ujjayi Breath

"*Ujjayi*" is Sanskrit for "victorious" or "to gain mastery." *Ujjayi* breath sounds like the ocean when it "inhales" coming into shore, and then "exhales," going back out to sea. This image of the ocean tide coming and going with your breath can help you stay focused on your breathing during your yoga practice.

### How to Create Ujjayi Breath

You develop your *Ujjayi* breath by constricting the back of your throat, like when you're about to whisper. *Which you are!* Except you're not going to whisper words, you're going to whisper your breath as you breathe your *Ujjayi* breath through your nose.

Breathe in, slowly and deeply, hear the ocean coming into the shore. There's a pause at the top of your breath, and then, slowly release your breath as the wave leaves the shore, returning out to the ocean. Then another pause at the bottom of your breath. Just like the tide, your breath returns again as it flows in and out through your nose.

*So relaxing and calming....*

### Ujjayi Breath with Your Yoga Movements

Here are a few of the reasons why it's good to use *Ujjayi* breath with your yoga movements:

*Ujjayi* breathing improves concentration during your practice. When you are absorbed in producing your ocean breath, you can remain in poses for longer periods.

*Ujjayi* breathing releases tension both physically and mentally.

*Ujjayi* breathing is meditative and deepens the mind-body-spirit connection that is central to yoga. It assists in grounding you and nurtures your self-awareness.

*Ujjayi* breathing promotes regulated heat for your body. The friction of the air as it passes through your lungs and throat generates internal body heat. This warmed air massages your internal organs, making stretching even more enjoyable, and the positions more readily achieved.

This generated internal heat helps your organs clear out toxins.

## *Ujjayi Breath and Your Health*
You may also discover that *Ujjayi* breath diminishes headaches, relieves sinus pressure, and decreases phlegm, all while providing strength for your nervous and digestive systems.

The full, deep, breath of *Ujjayi* breathing helps with the challenges of a yoga practice. As your breathing habit develops, you may discover that it helps with challenges elsewhere in your life as well.

The ancient yogis knew that there's an intimate connection between *breath* and *mind*. Your breath is a teacher. As you learn to pay attention to it, you'll learn much about yourself, encouraging equanimity and strength through all of life's passages.

# Nadi Shodhana – Alternate Nostril Breath

*Nadi Shodhana* comes from two Sanskrit words: *Nadi* = "flow" or "channel," and *Shodhana* = "purification." This breath exercise is focused on clearing the subtle channels of your body, mind, and spirit while balancing your masculine and feminine energies.

## How to Create Nadi Shodhana Breath

Sitting comfortably, keep your back, head, and neck in a straight line. Calmly take three or four deep breaths to become centered. Leave your left hand on your knee. Form the *Vishnu mudra* with your right hand by folding the index and middle fingers to your palm. Alternately, you may place your index and middle fingers between your eyebrows.

Inhale deeply, then with your right thumb, close off your right nostril. Exhale through your left nostril, picturing your breath traveling down the left side of your head, throat, down the left side of your spine through your organs, and down to your pelvic floor. Pause for a moment. Then inhale through your left nostril, picturing your breath traveling up from your pelvic floor up your left side, through all your organs, along the left side of your spine, and up into your throat and head. Pause.

Closing off your left nostril with your ring and pinky fingers, release your right nostril, and exhale, picturing your breath traveling down the right side of your head, throat, down the right side of your spine through your organs, and down to your pelvic floor. Pause. Then inhale through your right nostril, picturing your breath traveling up from your pelvic floor up your right side, through all your organs, along the right side of your spine, and up into your throat and head.

Continue this cycle for 20 or 30 breaths, then complete with an exhalation through your left nostril, relax your right hand in your lap or on your knee, and breathe deeply.

A variation is to count on the inhalation up to a comfortable number, for example, six, hold the breath for a count of two, then exhale for a count of six, and hold at the bottom of your breath for a count of two. An alternate discipline for this method is to increase the count on the exhalation and inhalation.

## *Nadi Shodhana Breath and Your Health*

*Nadi Shodhana* has many benefits. It removes toxins while infusing your body with oxygen. It reduces stress and anxiety. It clears your respiratory channels and helps to alleviate allergies. It calms and rejuvenates your nervous system.

*Nadi Shodhana* helps balance your hormones, aids mental clarity, and enhances concentration. It equalizes the right and left hemispheres of your brain, and your masculine-solar, and feminine-lunar, energies.

# Kapalabhati – Shining Skull Breath*

*Kapalabhati* comes from two Sanskrit words: *Kapala* = "skull" and *Bhati* = "light." When practicing *Kapalabhati*, many yogis experience a sensation of either literal light, or a feeling of lightness.

## How to Create Kapalabhati Breath

Sit in a comfortable position with your hands on your lower belly. Inhale deeply through your nose, and exhale deeply through your nose. Feel your lower belly expand in when you inhale and contract when you exhale. This requires that you breathe deeply into the depths of your core.

Inhale again and then exhale, contracting your lower belly sharply, with the breath forced out in a short burst. You will see your hands move in and out on your belly.

After the sharp exhale, your body will naturally inhale, passively. The attention is on the sharp, deep belly exhale. Keep your spine and shoulders still, the only movement is in your lower belly. Do this 20 times and pause, checking in with your body.

When first practicing *Kapalabhati* you may experience lightheadedness or slight dizziness. Progress slowly if you experience these symptoms, but the goal is to get up to 75 or 100 hundred repetitions. If you feel dizzy or become anxious, or your breath becomes strained, stop and breathe calmly.

Do the *Kapalabhati* breathing for no longer than a minute, then breathe deeply and exhale slowly as you calm into the quiet *Kapalabhati* produces.

## *Kapalabhati Breath and Your Health*

*Kapalabhati* is invigorating and warming. It tones and cleanses your lungs, sinuses, and your respiratory system by stimulating the release of toxins, while refreshing and rejuvenating your body, mind, and spirit.

Practiced regularly, *Kapalabhati* will strengthen your diaphragm and abdominal muscles. It increases your body's oxygen supply thus stimulating your brain, even as it calms the mind for meditation, or work that requires strong focus.

With practice, you will discover that *Kapalabhati*—and all yoga breathing exercises—brings balance into your life on physical, mental, emotional, and spiritual levels.

*Kapalabhati* is counter-indicated for people with high blood pressure, a hernia, or heart disease. Practice conservatively if you have asthma or emphysema, and stop if you're experiencing discomfort. The goal is to become more relaxed, and any breath exercise that generates tension is counterproductive to that goal.

What you think
You become.
Buddha

## *Favorite Yoga Routines*

One of the many wonderful aspects of yoga is that you can make it yours in any way that suits you best. Here you can write down sequences you've developed that let you completely relax, that empower you, that strengthen your body, that enhance your mind, and nurtures your spirit.

_____

_____

_____

_____

_____

_____

_____

_____

_____

_____

_____

_____

_____

_____

_____

_____

_____

_____

_____

_____

_____

_____

_____

# *Favorite Yoga Routines*

# *Favorite Yoga Routines*

_____
_____
_____
_____
_____
_____
_____
_____
_____
_____
_____
_____
_____
_____
_____
_____
_____
_____
_____
_____
_____
_____
_____
_____
_____
_____

# *Favorite Yoga Routines*

_____
_____
_____
_____
_____
_____
_____
_____
_____
_____
_____
_____
_____
_____
_____
_____
_____
_____
_____
_____
_____
_____
_____
_____
_____
_____

## *Disclaimer*

The information provided in this book is for educational and informational purposes and is not intended as a substitute for caring advice from your healthcare provider. Consult with your healthcare provider who knows your health profile before starting any exercise program.

## *My Gift for You ....*

As a thank you for reading *Chair Yoga – Easy, Healing Moves You Can Do with a Chair*, I have a gift for you, *Save Your Life with Stupendous Spices*. Download your ebook at the following link:

https://BookHip.com/DKHVDA

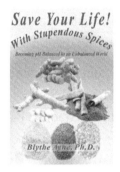

## *About the Author*

I live in the midst (and often the mist) of ten acres of forest, with domestic and wild creatures, where I create an ever-growing inventory of self-help, health, and meditation nonfiction books, fiction, short stories, and illustrated kid's books, along with quite a bit of poetry. I've also begun audio recording my books.

I do a bit of wood carving when I need a change of pace, and I'm frequently on a ladder, cleaning my gutters. It's spectacular being on a ladder … the vista opens up all around, and I feel rather like a bird or a squirrel, perched on a metal branch.

After I received my Doctorate from the University of California at Irvine in the School of Social Sciences, (majoring in psychology and ethnography), I moved to the Pacific Northwest to write and to have a modest private psychotherapy practice in a small town not much bigger than a village.

Finally, I decided it was time to put my full focus on my writing, where, through the world-shrinking internet, I could "meet" greater numbers of people. *Where I could meet you!*

All the creatures in my forest and I are glad you "stopped by." If you enjoyed **Chair Yoga – Easy, Healing Moves You Can Do with a Chair**, I hope you'll share the book with others.

If you want to write to me, I'd love to hear from you. Here's my email:

*Blythe@BlytheAyne.com*

And here's my website:

*www.BlytheAyne.com*

*And my Boutique of Books:*

*https://shop.BlytheAyne.com*

*I hope to "see" you again!*

*Blythe*

Mindfulness offers you
A present of the present.
Blythe Ayne

Made in the USA
Middletown, DE
01 July 2023

34357769R00066